YOGA BEYOND THE POSES

Bhakti YOGA

The Ultimate Beginner's Guide to Discover Bhakti Yoga, Yoga in Hinduism, and Bhagavad Gita!

Shreyanada Natha

Cover & design
Mattias Långström

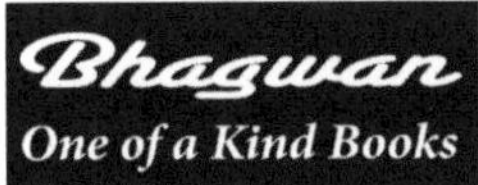

Bhagwan
One of a Kind Books

YOGA BEYOND THE POSES

Bhakti
YOGA

*The Ultimate Beginner's Guide
to Discover Bhakti Yoga, Yoga in Hinduism,
and Bhagavad Gita!*

Shreyanada Natha

ISBN 9789198839241

✳ ✳ ✳

2 FREE PREMIUM BONUS!

#1. *Download the **AUDIOBOOK** at the back of the book!*

#2. *Download **CHAKRA-INDEX IN COLOR** here!*

SCAN QR-CODE or go to:

https://bit.ly/47wdFVZ

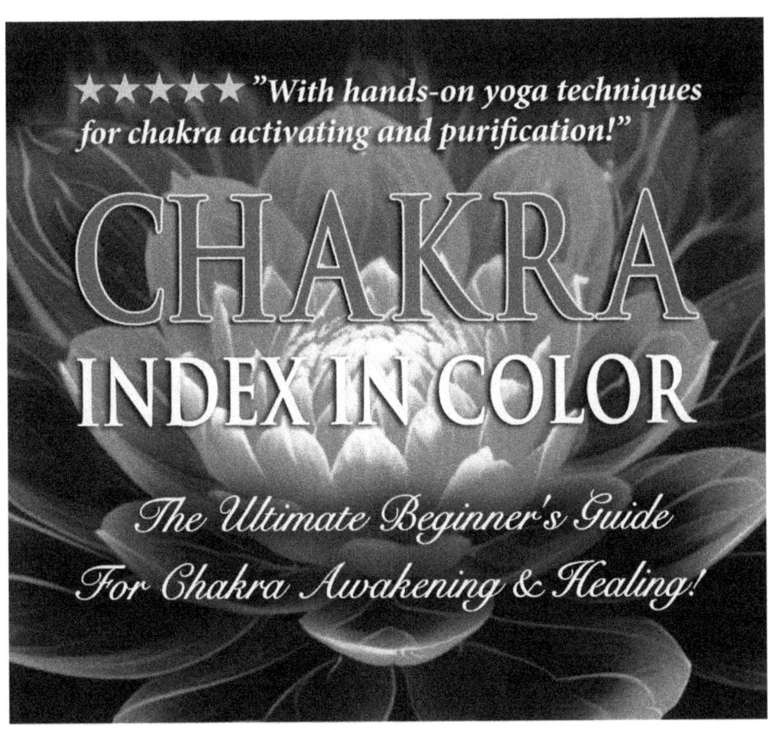

FREE PREMIUM Audiobook
Authentic Yoga Nidra Meditation – Manipura Chakra Awakening!

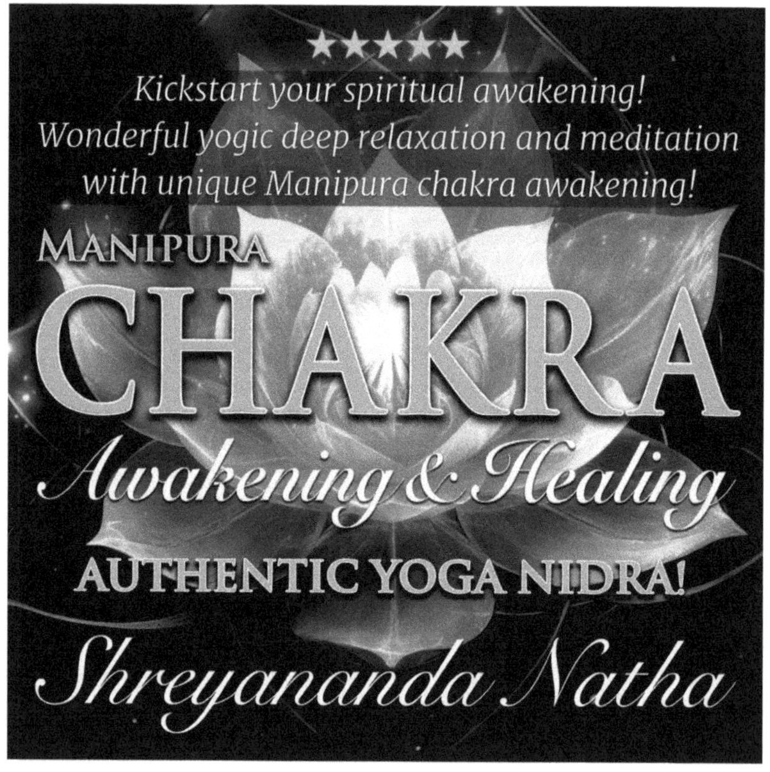

Download the **AUDIOBOOK** at the back of the book!

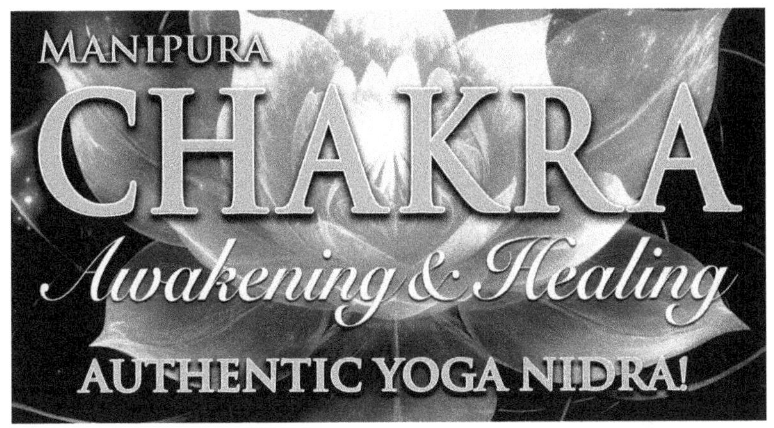

Kickstart your spiritual awakening! Wonderful yogic deep relaxation and meditation with unique Manipura chakra awakening and healing.

PRESENTATION

Yoga Nidra, or yogic sleep, is a unique meditation process that's powerfully profound and healing for body, mind, and spirit.

Practitioners are led into a state of deep relaxation and the experience of our chakra system.

Yoga Nidra offers extensive benefits, yet it is one of the most straightforward yoga practices.

All you have to do is put on your most comfortable clothes, find a quiet space, lie down on your back, and play the meditation.

**Yoga Beyond the Poses – Bhakti Yoga
The Ultimate Beginner's Guide to Discover Bhakti Yoga,
Yoga in Hinduism, and Bhagavad Gita!**
*Including A Premium Audiobook: Yoga Nidra Meditation –
Manipura Chakra Awakening And Healing!*

*The book describes yoga in Hinduism: Bhakti (the yoga of
love), Jnana and Karma yoga, and the Bhagavad Gita. Its
origin and mystery are from the ground up. It penetrates
deeply but remains easy to read, educational, and under-
standable. A must on the bookshelf for anyone interested
in Bhakti yoga – the yoga of love and who quickly wants to
know more.*

*The book is part of a series of seven yoga books, Yoga Beyond
the Poses: The Ultimate Beginner's Guide to Yoga, that delve
into the seven key areas of yoga.*

**INCLUDING A PREMIUM AUDIOBOOK:
AUTHENTIC YOGA NIDRA MEDITATION –
MANIPURA CHAKRA AWAKENING & HEALING!**
*Kickstart your spiritual awakening! Wonderful yogic deep
relaxation and meditation with unique Manipura chakra
awakening and healing.*

*Yoga Nidra, or yogic sleep, is a unique meditation process
that's powerfully profound and healing for body, mind, and*

spirit. Practitioners are led into a state of deep relaxation and the experience of our chakra system. Yoga Nidra offers extensive benefits, yet it is one of the most straightforward yoga practices. All you have to do is put on your most comfortable clothes, find a quiet space, lie down on your back, and play the meditation. –

Download the audiobook at the back of the book!

ABOUT THE BOOK SERIES
YOGA BEYOND THE POSES: *The Ultimate Beginner's Guide to Yoga!*

The book is part of a seven-book yoga series, Yoga Beyond the Poses: The Ultimate Beginner's Guide to Yoga, that delve into yoga's seven most important areas. They are straightforward to read, educational, and fascinating. A must on the bookshelf for anyone interested in yoga who quickly wants to know more.

MY NAME AND MY MISSION
Shreyananda Natha was the name I was given when I was initiated into the Natha Order and received the master mantra – the Shodasi mantra, after studying yoga and tantra for over twelve years, the highest mantra in yoga and tantra. It means "he who knows".

After practicing yoga and meditation continuously for over twenty years, having a yoga school for many years, and le-

*ading studies for yoga teachers, I wanted to get out more wi-
dely with yoga into our whole society, out of the small yoga
room. Spread the knowledge of yoga, our chakra system, and
Kundalini Shakti to anyone who will listen. What needed
to be added were educational fact books on yoga that didn't
just skim the surface or deal with the author's private life. So
it became my Sankalpa, my magical wish, and my mission
to create exciting yoga books that everyone should be able to
read and enjoy. To show how we can apply and use yoga in
different areas of life and achieve success and health. Here
and now.*

*If you like my books, feel free to follow me on my social
media, share and like, tell your friends about the books, and
write an honest review; one or two lines don't matter. All
support is precious.*

Thanks!

THE AUTHOR

Shreyananda Natha is the author of popular and best-selling yoga books. He has, among other things, written one of the most comprehensive books about yoga – EVERYTHING ABOUT YOGA and the study book – TEACHING YOGA AND MEDITATION BEYOND THE POSES. He is also a certified yoga and meditation teacher according to the EYTF international guidelines. He has undergone multi-year yoga teacher training under the guidance of Swami Omananda at Satyananda Ashram and holds the highest initiation in the tantric Natha order. He frequently travels to Asia and India to learn and gain knowledge and inspiration. He has immersed himself in tantric rituals and is known for his extensive knowledge of yoga, deep relaxation, and meditation.

"There is no authority that can say what yoga is. When you surrender yourself completely and fully and experience yoga without limitations and doubts, the true encounter with yoga occurs when you become one with the true experience within you. Only then will you understand what yoga is – for you. When you are no longer limited by neatness, shyness, and artificial thought patterns that act as a filter between you and the transformation. Yoga is a cultural-historical wealth still passed on from teacher to student and helps man find his way back to his true nature. It opens us up and attracts awareness. It strengthens our self-esteem, and our person's entire spectrum of possibilities suddenly becomes visible.

Yoga is not difficult or strange. You don't have to become a vegan, a monk, or be able to stand on your head. You just need to do your yoga regularly; the rest will take care of itself. You can use yoga and meditation to feel better, both physically and mentally, but also to achieve success and develop in all areas of life – here and now."

Good luck!

Namasté

I want to thank the teachers and students I've had over the years who have made my journey with yoga so enjoyable. Thank you for all the inspiration you have given me and for making this book possible. The yoga masters who no longer live among us – live on with each new person who immerses themselves in the yoga tradition.

Sri Swami Sivananda, Sri Swami Satyananda, Sri Tirumalai Krishnamacharya, Sri Swami Vishnudevananda, Sri K. Pattabhi Jois, Osho, Swami Nirdosha, Swami Omananda, Swami Janakananda, Ole Schmidt, Turiya, Maryam Abrishami and Sanna Kuittinen.

People who all searched for answers to what they sensed through an activated Ajna chakra. In yoga, they have learned the principles behind the universe, the collective consciousness, and the creative force, Kundalini Shakti. The duality behind everything, both what we see and what we don't see. Together, we are helped to pass on the previously secret knowledge about our gunas, nadis, and chakras to all who want to become a Rishi.

Aum Shri Durgayai Namaha

Shreyananda Natha

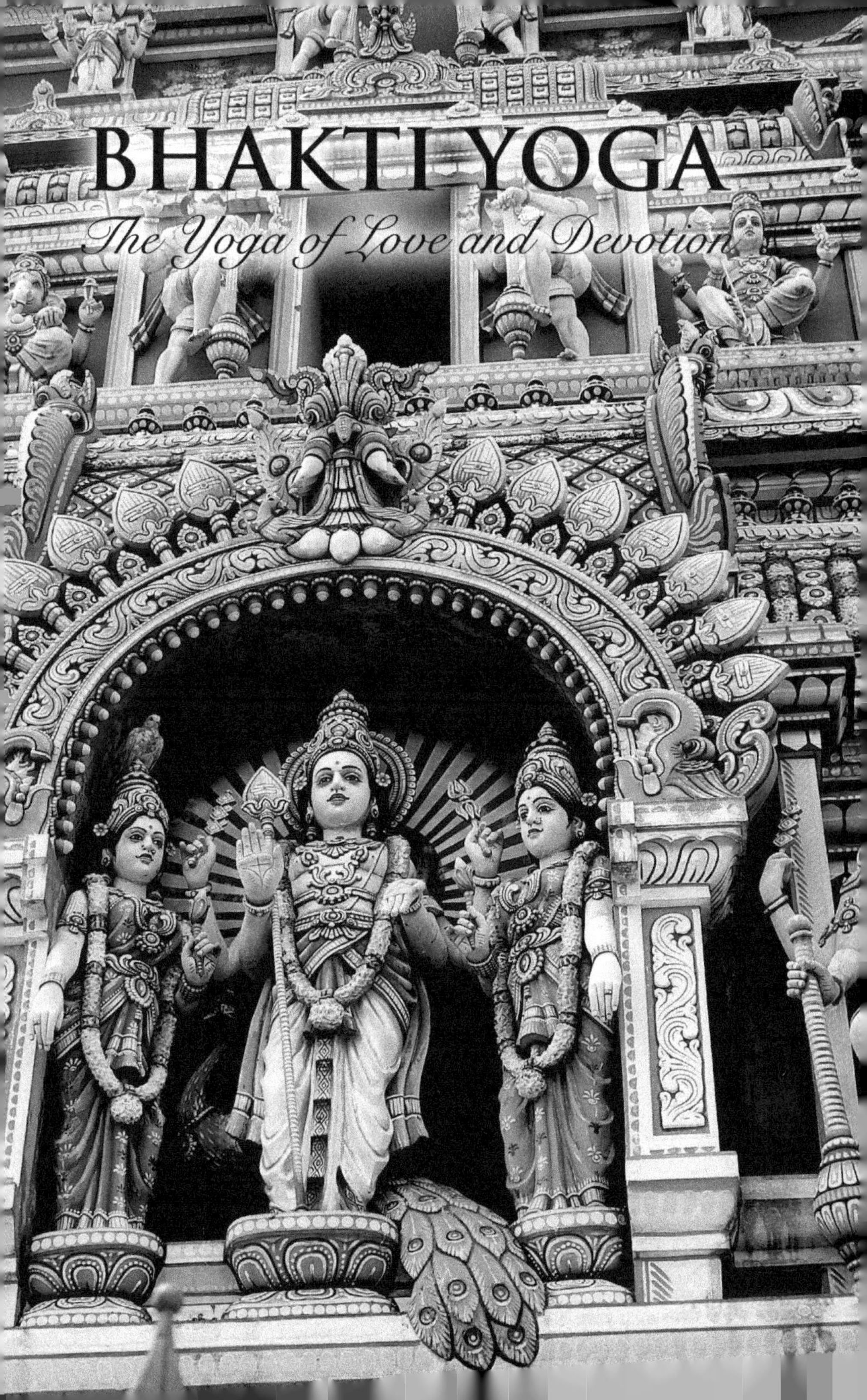
BHAKTI YOGA
The Yoga of Love and Devotion

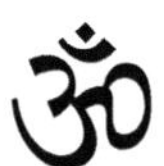

KARMA, BHAKTI & JNANA YOGA

HINDUISM

Hinduism differs from other religions in that it can be described as a collective name for a host of religious denominations that lack a common core. Most Hindus see Hinduism as a set of ritual acts, something practiced. But Hinduism is also a tradition that carries an extensive collection of knowledge – it is the religion with the most significant number of sacred texts.

In Hinduism, humans are perceived as thinking, biological, and social beings characterized by people's different interests and aptitudes for things. They worship different gods, read other texts, follow different teaching systems and gurus, and visit various temples. This view is the basis for the hierarchical method applied in Hinduism and the tolerance for each other's differences and diversity.

Diversity expresses the process of change and development that Prakriti undergoes. On the other hand, Purusha is what all individuals have in common – the unchanging self, the atman, as the Samkhya philosophy describes.

Samkhya and yoga both belong to the philosophical system

of Hinduism. The purpose of the systems is to guide man towards moksha, or freedom from the cycle of rebirth. Moksha is considered the fourth and final goal in a person's life.

The six philosophical systems are arranged in doctrinal pairs as follows:

Nyaya – logic.
Vaisheshika – atomic.

Samkhya – cosmic principle.
Yoga – Yoga.

Purva-Mimamsa (Vedanta) – ritual.
Uttara-Mimamsa (Vedanta) – theological.

The belief within these systems of a person's ability to be liberated differs from the bhakti-oriented theistic Vedan schools, whose adherents believe that a person depends on God's grace to be free from the cycle of rebirth.

Samkhya and yoga are described together in many of the Hindu texts, indicating an early connection to each other.

The Katha, Svetasvatara, and Maitri Upanishads describe yogic exercises and Samkhya together. In the Katha Upanishad, yoga is used as a means of meditation. Yoga and Samk-

hya are also mentioned in close connection in the Mahabharata. Here, the goal of yoga is described as the realization of the atman (the self) and Brahman (matter).

The Bhagavad Gita, part of the Mahabharata, describes yoga in three ways – Jnana, Karma, and Bhakti yoga. Krishna is seen here as the master of yoga.

The Yoga Sutras of Patanjali, an essential text in Hinduism and the most important work of classical yoga, has become and serve as a basic description. Here, too, Samkhya plays a central role. Even yoga traditions that do not share the same view of the ultimate reality have embraced the Yoga Sutras, which describe them logically and coherently. In the Yoga Sutras, yoga is defined as the cessation of the mind's activities, which we today call meditation.

DHARMA

A central concept in Hinduism is dharma, likened to duty, law, rightness, and firmness. Many Hindus today call their religion Sanatana dharma (the eternal dharma). Dharma is the eternal order, and in the oldest scriptures, it refers to the various rituals and duties performed to maintain social and cosmic order.

Dharma is based on the notion that humans maintain the universe through actions. Various rituals, civil and crimi-

nal law, stages of life, pilgrimages, sacrifices, etc, cover these actions. Dharma is used to structure society and the life of the individual. It plays a significant role in the caste systems applied in Hindu culture.

Following one's dharma should lead to a better rebirth and be a path to ultimate salvation.

TRADITIONS

The core tradition of Hinduism is Brahmanical, the most dominant and widespread practice in India. Men in the tradition are authoritarian. The Vedic texts play a central role and are seen as revelations. The tradition includes the priesthood, a sacred language (Sanskrit), and the perception of a holy social order. Rituals are performed in temples and ceremonies in the home. Hindu deities such as Shiva, Vishnu, Rama, Krishna, Durga, Kali, and Ganesha are worshipped. Pilgrimages, festivals, rules about food, and cleanliness are also important.

The other primary focus is organizations, where the focus is usually on moksha (salvation). These typically have a founder, and some are more ritually oriented (Sri Vishnuism and Sri Vidya), while others function as organizations for ascetics (Vishnuite: Ramanandi and Nada; or Shivaite: Natha and Aghori). They are often bearers of different yoga traditions, and men from the Brahmin class are often seen as leaders of these groups.

The guru movements also belong to this tradition; these often have to compete for followers. Many have also succeeded in communicating their teachings internationally, such as Maharishi Mahesh Yogi (Transcendental Meditation) and A.C. Bhaktivedanta Swami Prabhupada (International Society for Krishna Consciousness).

A third focus is the village and tribe-based traditions of India. Priests in this tradition are not from the Brahmin class, and gods with a local connection are worshipped. The Brahmin core tradition sees these practices as unclean, which has led to a tense relationship.

VISHNUISM, SHIVAISM AND SHAKTISM

Sacrifice rituals were a central part of the Brahmanic tradition but became less important as the ascetic ideology emerged. Knowledge and renunciation became more critical than being freed from the cycle of rebirth. Many influential gods in the Vedic sacrificial tradition fell away, while Shiva and Vishnu remained important. Groups sprang up where one of these gods was worshipped, laying the foundation for Hinduism. The ritual worship of gods (puja) that then arose competed with the sacrificial culture (yajna).

Seventy percent of Hindus worship Vishnu or one of his avatars, such as Rama or Krishna. Vishnu's task is to sustain the world. In the form of Krishna, he evokes feelings of love and care. In the form of Rama, he symbolizes the world order, dharma, and the dutiful man. Worship and devotion to a personal god is what characterizes Vishnuism. Still, there are also organizations for ascetics, and some groups have taken up some tantrism and instead worshipped a goddess such as Lakshmi.

Twenty-eight percent of Hindus worship Shiva, his family members, his wife Parvati, and their sons Ganesha and Skanda. Shiva is a great yogi and a friendly god, but he also has sides where he appears dangerous, destructive, and terrible. Shivaism is expected in the Himalayan region and is mainly yogic. Some Hindu ascetics also worship him.

The 13th to 16th centuries were an excellent time for Shivaite ascetics and Natha yogis in northern India. They practiced Hatha yoga and various tantric rituals. Gorakhnatha is the most famous Natha yogi. He was a student of Matsyendranatha, a disciple of Siva. Through Hatha yoga, one could stop the body's decay and activate kundalini Shakti to create an immortal body leading to the Shiva state. According to Natha yogis, only Hatha yoga could lead to this condition; other religious paths were considered unnecessary.

About two percent of Hindus follow Shaktism and worship the goddess Shakti, the female power of the supreme divine principle. She is seen as the ultimate reality (Brahman), the

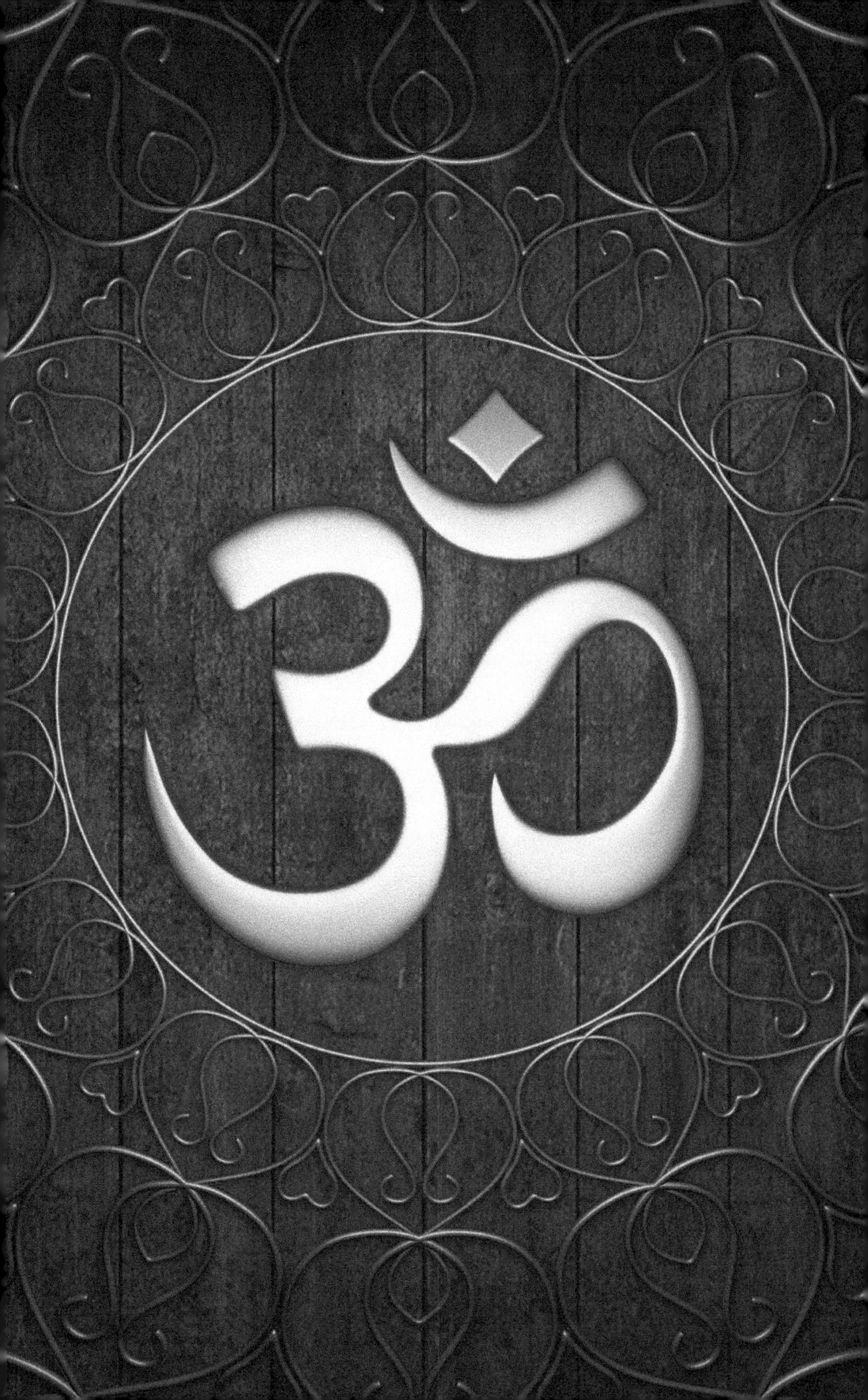

creative force (Shakti), the matter in creation (Prakriti), the one who hides (Maya), and the savior. Shaktism has evolved from Shivaism. Many female figures were found during the excavations in the Indus Valley, although it is unclear what they represented. In the seventh century A.D., Shaktism was mentioned in the written traditions.

Female ideology also plays a central role in tantrism, whose concept is based on the belief that our external environment and bodies consist of both female and male aspects and that salvation comes through uniting this polarity. To achieve tantric salvation (sadhana), mantras, mudras, nyasa, and puja are used. Tantrism combines Jnana and Karma yoga. Knowledge ultimately saves a person, and action gives them experience of the ultimate reality. Kundalini yoga was developed as a separate branch of yoga within tantrism and is based on the goddess ideology of tantrism and Shaktism. The path of tantrism is the most effective for the world we live in today, the Kali era. Old techniques are more challenging to apply.

HINDUISM AND YOGA

In the 1920s, archaeological excavations along the Indus River uncovered the remains of two large cities, Mohenjo Daro and Harappa. Both yoga and Hinduism most likely originated from this era, when the Indus and Saraswati civilizations existed.

The excavations also uncovered fall stones, an essential symbol of the God Shiva, and signets, one of which depicted a person with animal horns sitting in a meditation position surrounded by four animals. Shiva is often called the master of animals, which may indicate that he was already being worshipped when the Indus culture flourished between 5,000 and 3,000 BC. Shiva is called the great yogi, suggesting that yoga originated from this time.

Modern technology has helped establish that the Saraswati River dried up sometime in the 30th century B.C. The river Saraswati is praised in the Rigveda, suggesting this sacred text must have come into being earlier. Yoga is mentioned in the Rigveda, indicating that it originated before the 30th century B.C.

Yoga is central to Hinduism and a physical and mental discipline to achieve spiritual salvation. Most people have experienced this part of Hinduism – both Hindus and non-Hindus. The original goal of yoga in the Hindu tradition is to reach salvation or enlightenment with the help of the body, using various physical and mental techniques. In the West, yoga has been chiefly used to strengthen the body and find peace. Like Hinduism, yoga is pluralistic, meaning many physical and mental exercises depend on your chosen tradition.

Traditions can define the concept of yoga in different ways. The most common translation among Hindus is "union," which refers to a union between body and soul. The Patanjali Yoga Sutras, one of the most essential texts in yoga, defines yoga chitta vritti nirodhah, or cessation of the activities of the mind.

Within the yoga traditions, the term yoga has five primary meanings:

1. A disciplined method of achieving a goal.

2. A technique for controlling the body.

3. A name for one of the six philosophical systems of Hinduism.

4. Combined with words such as Hatha, mantra, and laya, yoga refers to traditions focusing on specific yoga techniques.

5. Objectives for the practice of yoga.

Central to any tradition is breathing and breath control. Holding the breath is considered a ritual act in the Brahmanic tradition. Atharvaveda tells of breathing and its connection to the body's energies. The Chandogya Upanishad describes five different types of breathing: inner sound, and nadis.

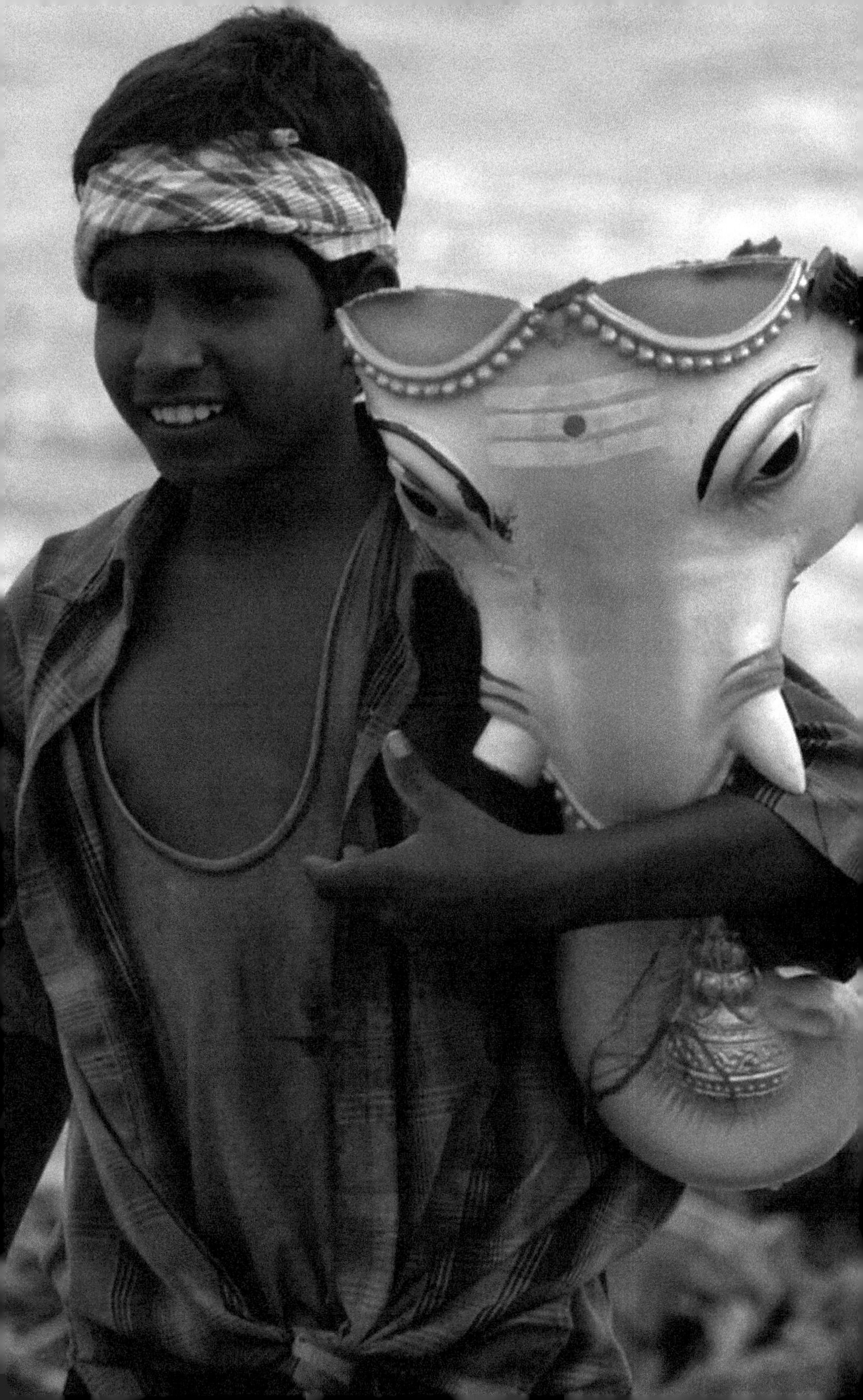

YOGA AND BUDDHISM

Buddhism has its roots in Indian yoga and was, from its beginning, a form of yoga. Yoga teachers taught the Buddha himself, and his experiences became the basis of the Buddhist meditation doctrine. Buddhists and Hindu yoga are thus closely related and may have influenced each other for hundreds of years. Concepts such as nirodha/nirvana (cessation) and dukkha (suffering) are expected in both traditions. The Buddhist eight-fold path and Indian eight-fold yoga have many similarities. The big difference is that in Indian yoga, the body and breathing have a much greater significance. The most crucial goal in both traditions is to end avidya, false knowledge.

THE SCRIPTURES OF VEDA

Veda means knowledge, and the scriptures are divided into four parts (Samantha):

1. The Rigveda (roughly the 30th century B.C.) is the oldest part of the Vedic scriptures, where yoga and the Saraswati river are mentioned. These Vedas are recited hymns and serve as regulations for various rituals. Different yoga techniques were developed to strengthen the ability to concentrate to perform the ceremonies successfully.

2. The Samaveda are Vedas with sung hymns.

3. The Yajurveda are Vedas with ritual texts.

4. The Atharvaveda are Vedas with magic formulas.

According to the Vedic worldview, our world reflects the cosmic world. One can create a harmonious existence by maintaining the heavenly order on our planet. To get an inner picture of the cosmic order, followers use yoga techniques such as regulated breathing, mantra singing, and concentration exercises.

These smiths are the first part of the wood. Three more texts are included:

1. Brahmana: comments on the vedas that explain the rituals of each samitha.

2. Aranyaka: "Forest books".

3. The Upanishads: The last part of the Vedas and often seen as the most important. This esoteric text describes the worldview in Vedanta, India's most famous philosophical system.

The Upanishads are based on four fundamental concepts:

1. The Brahman (world soul) is identical to the atman (the human soul), which means that the creative energy of the universe is similar to our inner self.

2. The realization that the unity of everything leads to spiritual enlightenment – moksha. This insight frees us from the cycle of rebirth.

3. The law of karma means that our thoughts and actions affect our future.

4. You are born according to your karma if you do not reach insight.

In the Katha, Svetasvarata, and Maitri Upanishads, you can find descriptions of yoga exercises and Samkhya concepts and performances, indicating that yoga has been associated with Samkhya from an early age.

"IT IS THE HIGHEST STATE:
WHEN THE FIVE SENSE ORGANS
AND THE MIND HAVE CALMED DOWN,
AND THE INTELLECT IS IMMOBILE.
THEY CALL THIS CONTROL OF THE SENSES
YOGA.
THEN HE IS FREE FROM DISTURBANCES,
FOR YOGA IS BOTH ORIGIN AND CESSATION."

(KATHA-UPANISHAD 6.10-11)

"By holding the body with its top three parts right and getting the feelings and senses to go in the heart, the sage crosses all dangerous rivers with Brahman as a boat.

While controlling breathing and all movements, he should breathe through his nose with manipulated breathing sounds, the wise control his mind as he steers a chariot drawn by wild horses.

In an even and clean place, free from pebbles, fire, and sand, near running water, in one location the mind finds attractive and to which the eye does not react as ugly, in a hidden area sheltered from the wind, he should practice yoga."

(Svetasvatara-upanishad 2.8-2.10)

THE MAHABHARATA

Yoga is also mentioned in the Mahabharata, which belongs to the category of itihasa (history) and which is one of two great epic works in Hinduism, especially in Books 12 and 13, where yoga is described in close connection with Samkhya.

"WHAT YOGIS SEE IS THE SAME AS
THE FOLLOWERS OF SAMKHYA PERCEIVE.
HE IS A SAGE WHO SEES SAMKHYA AND YOGA
AS THE SAME."

(MAHABHARATA 12.293.30)

The Bhagavad Gita is a mythological work of poetry and the most crucial scripture in Bhakti yoga. This great epic belongs to the Mahabharata and was added about 700 AD. It is seen as a summary of the Upanishads. Here, Krishna is described as the master of yoga, which is seen as a disciplined method of achieving a goal. Three yoga paths are described – Jnana, Karma, and Bhakti, of which Bhakti is considered the highest.

"IT IS BETTER TO FOLLOW ONE'S DHARMA
BADLY THAN ANOTHER'S FLAWLESSLY."

(BHAGAVAD GITA 3.35)

"WHILE SITTING THERE,
HE SHOULD PRACTICE YOGA
TO CLEAR THE MIND,
KEEP THE MIND ATTACHED TO AN OBJECT,
AND RESTRAIN THE MIND
AND EMOTIONS ACTIVITY."

(BHAGAVAD GITA 6.12)

DIFFERENT YOGA PATHS

As said, yoga is a broad tradition with many branches and techniques. Down the ages, masters have developed various methods for spiritual enlightenment. There are no direct boundaries between the yoga paths, but everyone goes in some way into each. Within a yoga tradition, one can use many different techniques.

KARMA YOGA – THE WAY OF ACTION

Karma yoga is a way of action and is mainly suitable for outgoing people. It means working, performing social activities, and helping others without expecting anything. Karma yoga continues the Vedic sacrificial doctrine, where sacrifices were made to the gods. In the Bhagavad Gita, sacrificial acts mean one is loyal to the warning doctrine that they follow their dharma and the class they belong to.

Today, Karma yoga is more about selfless, moral action. The job itself is not the most important; one's attitude during its execution is. One's mood determines whether the activity or job is perceived as liberating or binding, painful and challenging. Whatever you choose to do, make sure you always do your best. If you can do the job better, you do it. One should not let negative thoughts, such as fear of criticism, hold one back. You should also feel free of your job but be prepared to leave it if necessary. Mahatma Gandhi are a famous Karma yogi.

BHAKTI YOGA – THE WAY OF DEDICATION

This path is suitable for people who are emotional with nature. One surrenders oneself to God through prayers, worship, and rituals, driven by the power of love and experiencing God as love itself. Being devoted and loving towards a personal god is considered to lead to salvation. Chanting and singing God's name is a central part of Bhakti yoga.

RAJA YOGA – THE WAY OF MEDITATION

Often called the royal way, Raja yoga involves the control of thoughts. One trains the mind through meditation and transforms mental and physical energy into spiritual energy. Raja yoga is also called Ashtanga yoga, which refers to "eight-step yoga," which should systematically lead to control of the mind. Meditation takes place by itself when the body and energy are under control and in harmony.

Ashtanga yoga's eight steps – the Yoga Sutras of Patanjali:

1. Yamas – five basic ideas about moral discipline, "do not do":
Ahimsa – do not use violence.
Sathyam – be authentic.
Brahmacharya – moderation, control over desire, chastity.
Asteya – do not steal.
Aparighara – do not be greedy.

2. Niyamas – five basic ideas about ethical action, "should do":

Saucha – external and internal cleanliness, such as thoughts, speech, and hygiene.
Santosha – contentment.
Tapas – restraint, self-discipline.
Swadhyaya – studies.
Ishvara pranidhana – the worship of God.

3. Asana – body position.
The lotus position. To be able to sit utterly immobile so as not to be distracted by the physical body during meditation.

4. Pranayamas – controlled breathing.
Controlled breathing to control the prana in the body, which calms the mind.

5. Pratyahara – directs the sense organs inward.
It calms the mind when not disturbed by the environment and external stimuli.

6. Dharana – concentration.
Concentration is achieved by focusing on an object.

7. Dhyana – meditation.
After a long period of concentration, meditation is achieved.

8. Samadhi – ecstasy.
Prolonged meditation leads to ecstasy. The yogi becomes at one with the object of meditation when the movements of the mind cease.

JNANA YOGA – THE WAY OF KNOWLEDGE

This path is the most challenging because it requires a strong will and sharp intellect. It is suitable for theoretically inclined people. A Jnana yogi understands the transient and the eternal in life by studying Vedanta, which belongs to the Upanishads, the last part of the Vedic scriptures. It is challenging to reach spiritual insight through theoretical knowledge; therefore, it is essential to practice other yoga paths as a preparation. Ramana Maharishi is a well-known Jnana yogi.

THE MANTRA

The mantra consists of words and syllables that carry a unique vibration and affect the mind and body in a positive and strengthening way. According to tradition, mantras have been used to reach a deeper plane of consciousness.

With mantra meditation, you calm your thoughts and mind. Repeating the same mantra repeatedly does not give the mind any new stimulus; instead, it allows the subconscious mind to wake up. Old thoughts and memories have an opportunity to come to the surface, and the subconscious mind can be purified from them. One looks more clearly at life and is no longer governed by old thought patterns. In the same way that asanas are meant to strengthen and purify the body, the mantra is meant to calm and "clean up" the mind.

In yoga, it is believed that everything in the universe consists of energy that vibrates differently. Mantras are high vibrations that should benefit and positively affect our bodies. When we recite or sing a mantra, we begin to vibrate at the same rate. Our palate has eighty-four meridian points that affect the pituitary gland, the pineal gland, and the brain's chemical balance. When we pronounce specific mantras, the tongue hits these meridian points, which can increase mental clarity and awareness.

Most often, one recites a mantra one hundred and eight times. Our physical and subtle body has seventy-two thousand energy channels called nadis. One hundred and eight meet at Hrit padma, the area around the Anahata chakra. By repeating a mantra one hundred and eight times, the whole physical and subtle body is permeated by its energy.

THE GAYATRI MANTRA

The gayatri mantra is said to be the oldest mantra, with its origins in the Rigveda Vedic scripture. It is sometimes called savitri because, in the mantra, one prays to Deva Savitr, the sun god who was worshipped during the Vedic period (the sun before sunrise is called savitri and after sunrise surya).

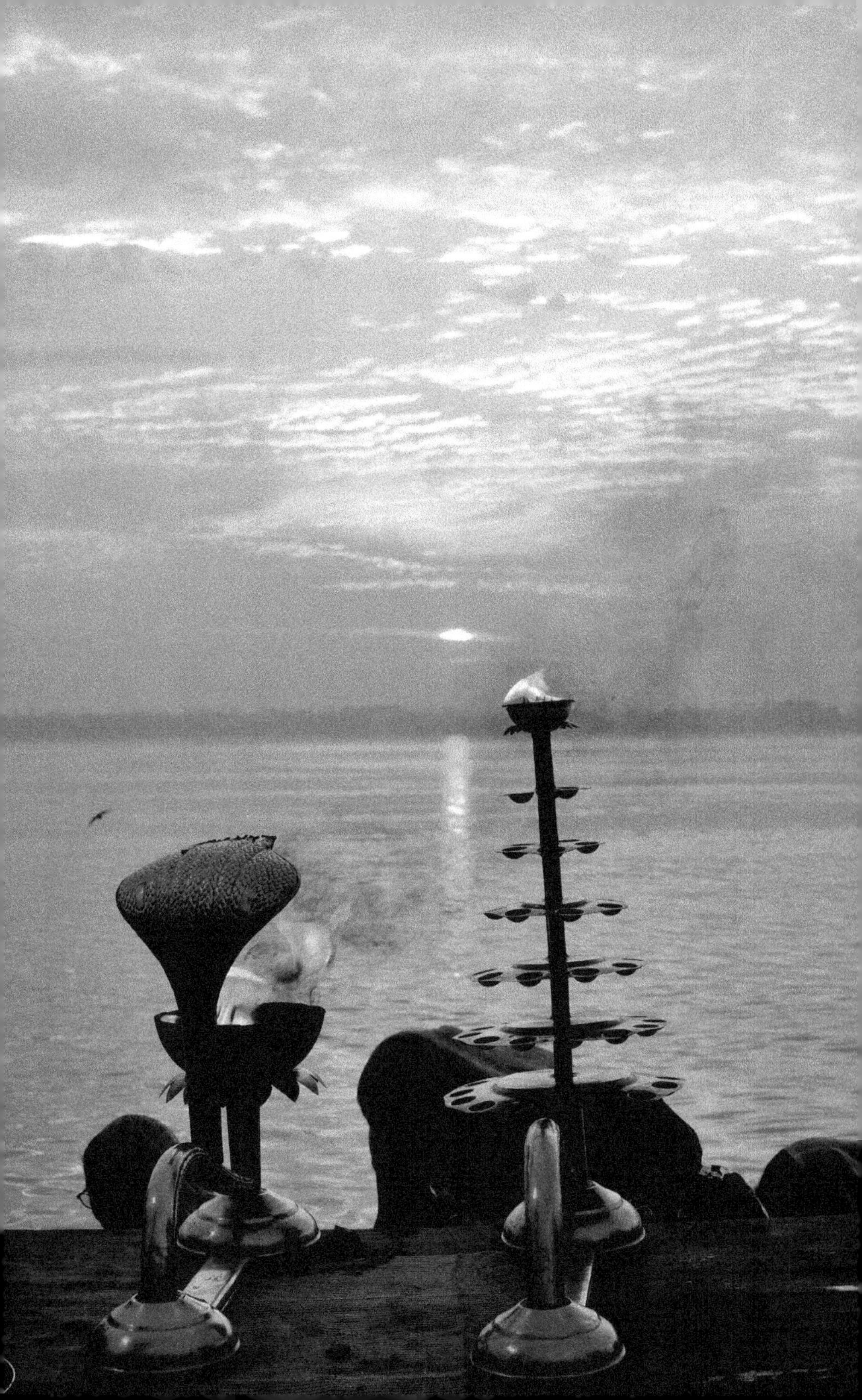

The gayatri mantra is also found in other Hindu texts, such as the Bhagavad Gita, and is essential in Hindu traditions. It is taught to children when they turn eight years old.

The gayatri mantra is said to heal physically, mentally, and emotionally. It expands consciousness, promotes spiritual development, and develops intellectual potential, knowledge, and wisdom. It seems sattvic.

THE GAYATRI MANTRA

Om bhur bhuvaha svaha
Tat savitur varenyam
Bhargo devasya dhimahi
Dhiyo yonah prachodayat

"Praise to the source of all things.
It is due to you that we attain true
happiness on the planes of earth,
astral, casual. It is due to your
transcendent nature that you are
worthy of being worshiped and
adored. Ignite us with your
all-pervading light."

THE MAHAMRITYUNJAYA MANTRA

This mantra is also rooted in the Rigveda Vedic literature and is called the tryambakam mantra. It is dedicated to "the three-eyed," an epithet of Rudra, who was later characterized as Shiva.

The mahamrityunjaya mantra provides peace and protection. It is said to heal physically, mentally, and emotionally. It counteracts rajas.

THE MAHAMRITYUNJAYA MANTRA

Om triambakam yajamahe
Sugandhim pushti vardanam
Urvarukamiva bandhanan
Mrityor muksheeya mamritat

"Shelter me, the three-eyed Lord Shiva. Bless me with health and immortality and sever me from the clutches of death, even as a cucumber is cut from its creeper."

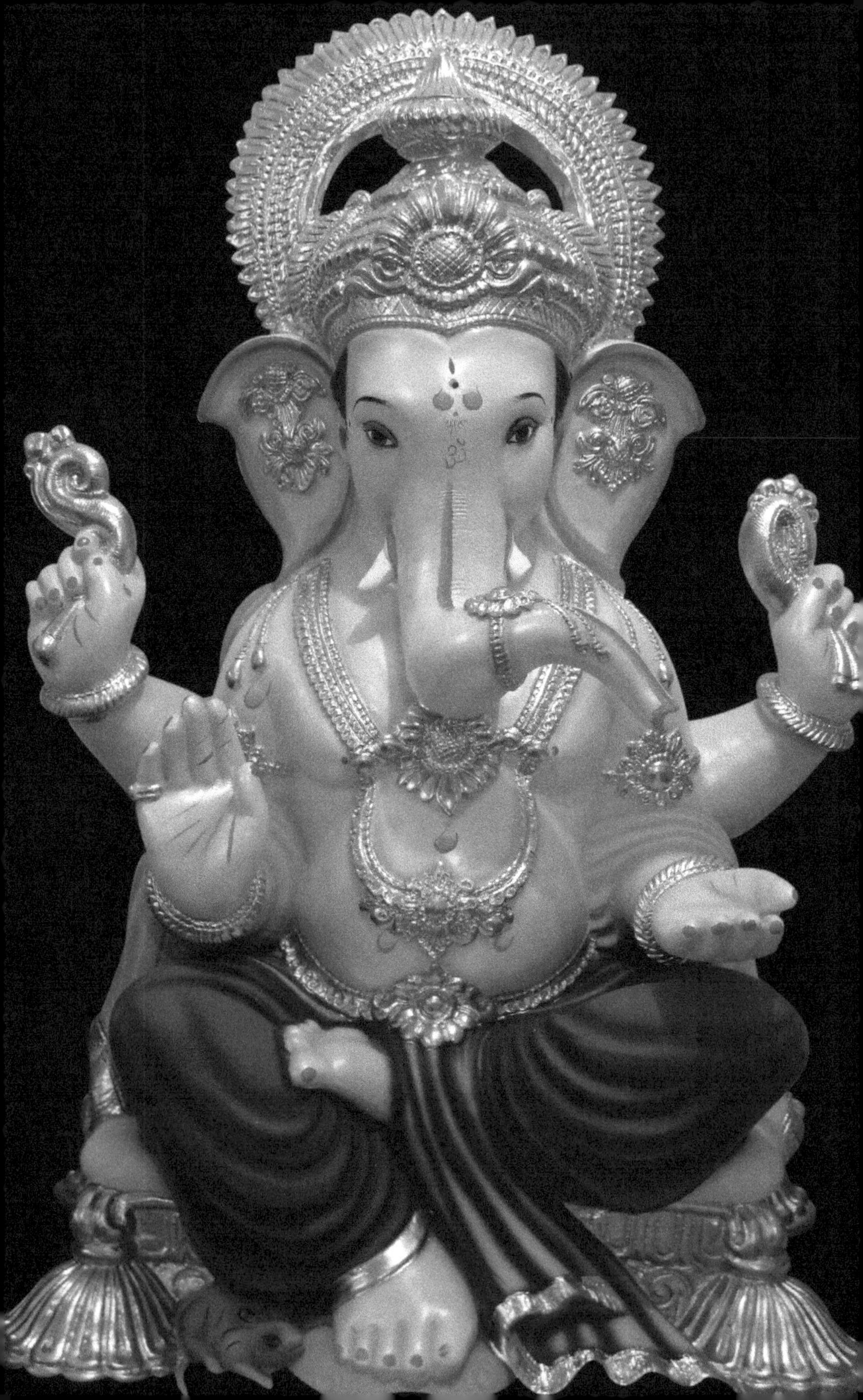

THE INFLUENCE OF TANTRISM ON YOGA

During the post-classical period, it was primarily tantrism that influenced the yoga tradition.

According to tantrism, the human body's divine power (Kundalini Shakti) is inactive. This brings the physical body into focus for the ritual exercises, a new phenomenon in the spiritual history of India.

THE BHAGAVAD GITA

The Bhagavad Gita (the "Song of God") is the god Krishna's song. It is a mythological work in Sanskrit and an independent story in the great Mahabharata epic. In the Bhagavad Gita, a dialogue occurs between Krishna and Prince Arjuna just before the great battle of Kurukshetra. Arjuna faces a dilemma: his duty as a warrior is to follow his dharma and begin the war, but at the same time, he sees it as a terrible sin to kill the many great men, relatives, and gurus in the opponents' army. To accompany the prince through this challenging decision, Krishna teaches him various forms of yoga. The story takes place about five thousand years ago.

The Bhagavad Gita can be seen as a summary of the Upanishads. Each chapter ends with the Bhagavad Gita being called Upanishad.

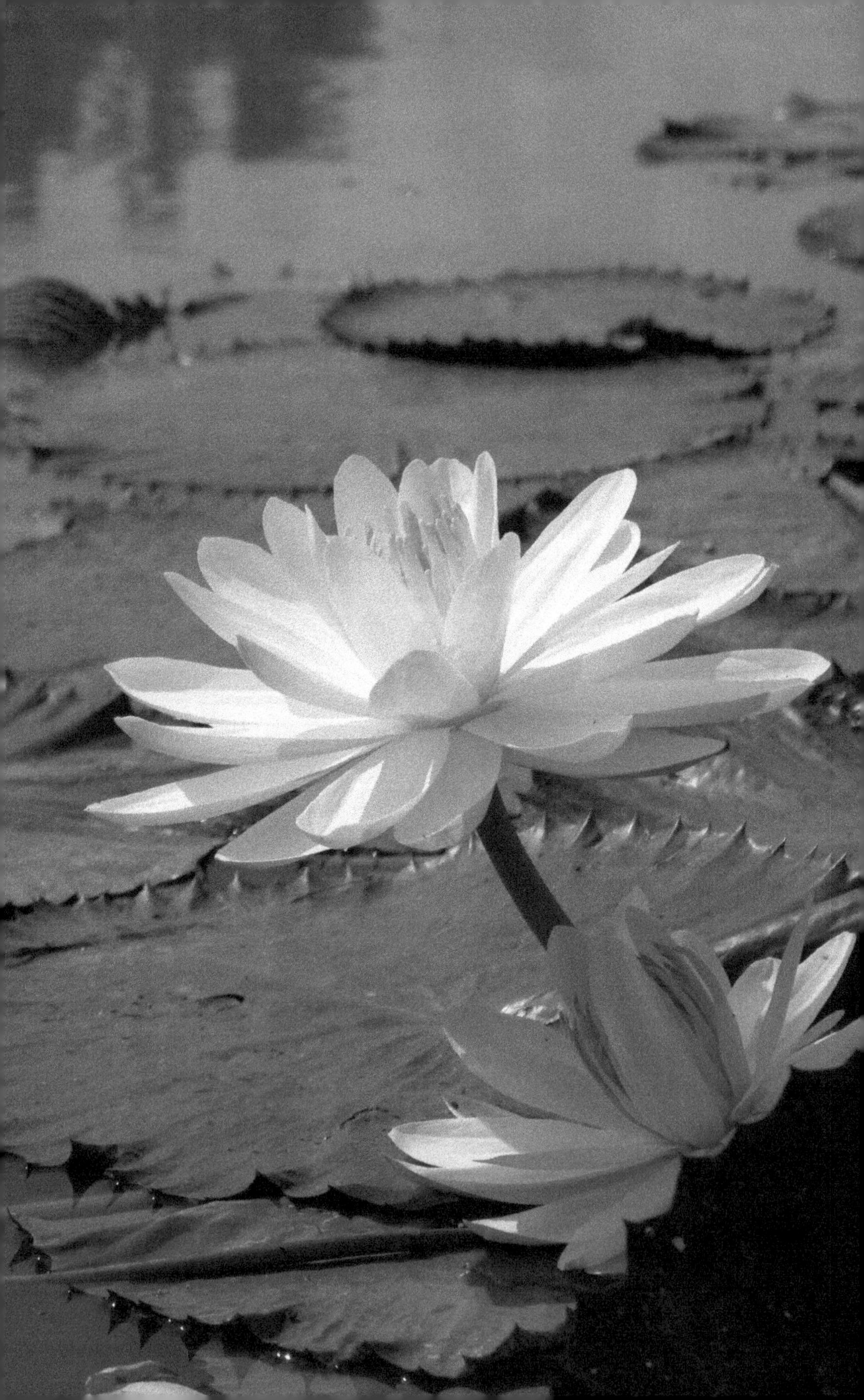

Krishna says in Bhagavad Gita 3.3 that there have been two paths since ancient times:

Karma yoga – the way of action, to do one's duty without worrying about the outcome.

Jnana yoga – the way of knowledge, knowledge of the self (atman).

Other ways are variants of these.

Krishna shows his vishvarupa, his universal form, for Arjuna on the battlefield at Kurukshetra.

The Bhagavad Gita consists of eighteen chapters:

1. Arjuna lets Krishna pull his chariot to a place in the middle of the two armies. When Arjuna sees his relatives on the opposite side of Kurus, he loses motivation and decides not to fight.

2. Krishna explains to Arjuna that his concern about fighting against his relatives and gurus is unjustified because only the body can be killed, while the eternal self is immortal. Krishna reminds Arjuna to follow his dharma and wage war as a warrior.

3. Arjuna asks why he has to fight if knowledge is more important than action. Krishna emphasizes that the right way to act is to carry out one's duties for good without clinging to the results.

4. Krishna says he has lived through many births and always taught yoga to protect the righteous and annihilate the unrighteous. He emphasizes the importance of trusting a guru.

5. Arjuna asks Krishna if it is better to refrain from action or to perform actions. Krishna replies that both ways can be good, but that action, Karma yoga, is the highest.

6. Krishna describes the correct position of meditation and the process of achieving samadhi.

7. Krishna teaches the way of knowledge, Jnana yoga.

8. Krishna defines the terms Brahman, dharma, karma, atman, adhibhuta, and adhidaiva and explains how to remember him at the moment of death and attain a higher state.

9. Krishna describes panentheism, "all beings are in me," as a way of remembering him in all circumstances.

10. Krishna declares that he is the ultimate source of all ma-

terial and spiritual worlds. Arjuna recognizes Krishna as the supreme being and quotes famous scholars who have done the same.

11. At Arjuna's request, Krishna demonstrates a theophany, its "universal form," Visvarupa: a terrifying creature that is turned in all directions at the same time, which spreads the radiation from a thousand suns around it, and which contains all other beings and all matter that exists.

12. Krishna describes the process of devotion, Bhakti yoga.

13. Krishna describes matter (Prakriti) and consciousness (purusha).

14. Krishna talks about the three states, gunas, constituting all beings.

15. Krishna describes a symbolic tree, representing material existence, its roots in heaven, and its foliage on earth. He explains that this tree should be felled with the "axe of indifference" so that one can move on to a higher state.

16. Krishna describes the human traits of divine and demonic beings. He advises that the higher state can be achieved by renouncing lust, anger, and greed and distinguishing right actions from wrong deeds through buddhi and advice from scriptures, thereby acting right.

17. Krishna talks about the three variants of faith, knowledge, actions, and eating habits linked to the three gunas.

18. Krishna asks Arjuna to abandon all dharma and submit to him. He describes this as the ultimate and final perfection of life.

Did you like the book? Feel free to follow me on my social media, share and like, tell your friends about the books, and feel free to write an honest review; one or two lines don't matter. All support is precious. Thanks!

On my Facebook page and Instagram, I post exciting news and tips on temporary offers and benefits you can take advantage of. I often also post my yoga routine and other things related to nutrition and health that may be interesting to take part in. So feel free to join them so you don't miss anything interesting:

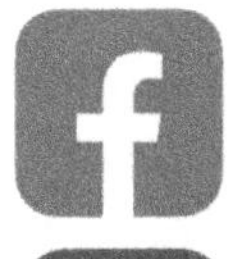 *facebook.com/bhagwanoneofakindbooks*

 *instagram.com/bhagwanoneofakindbooks/*

MY BOOKS AND BOOK SERIES

I have two book series that have different audiences. Great Yoga Books – is a series with the most comprehensive fact books on yoga for those who want to explore the subject in depth. Here, you will also find classic yoga books that are rarely translated, such as Patanjali's Yoga Sutras and Hatha Yoga Pradipika. My second series, Yoga Beyond the Poses: The Ultimate Beginner's Guide to Yoga, covers one yoga topic at a time and is extra easy to read with larger text. For those who find it challenging to read extensive books and want a good and broad overview of the subject quickly. Both series are also available as audiobooks.

★★★★★

TEACHING YOGA
&
MEDITATION
BEYOND
THE POSES

BESTSELLING AUTHOR

Shreyananda Natha

Teaching Yoga and Meditation Beyond the Poses – A unique and practical workbook!

Teaching Yoga and Meditation Beyond the Poses – A unique and practical workbook for aspiring yoga teachers who want to teach yoga and meditation beyond the poses.

Teaching Yoga and Meditation Beyond the Poses is a unique and essential resource for new and experienced teachers and a guide for all yoga students interested in refining their skills and knowledge. Teaching Yoga and Meditation is also ideal as a core textbook in yoga teacher training programs.

The book covers fundamental yoga philosophy and history topics, including a historical presentation of classical yoga literature: Yoga Sutras of Patanjali, Bhagavad Gita, etc. Each of the seven major styles of yoga is described, from Hatha yoga, Raja yoga, Tantra yoga, Bhakti yoga, and Kundalini yoga, to knowledge about the chakras, Ayurveda and magic mantras and yantras. The book provides extensive support and tools for teaching integrated and classical yoga (asanas), breathing techniques (pranayama), deep relaxation (Yoga Nidra), and meditation (Ajapa Japa). The book is divided into eight modules with associated knowledge tests and complete yoga and meditation classes.

https://rb.gy/9s6edj

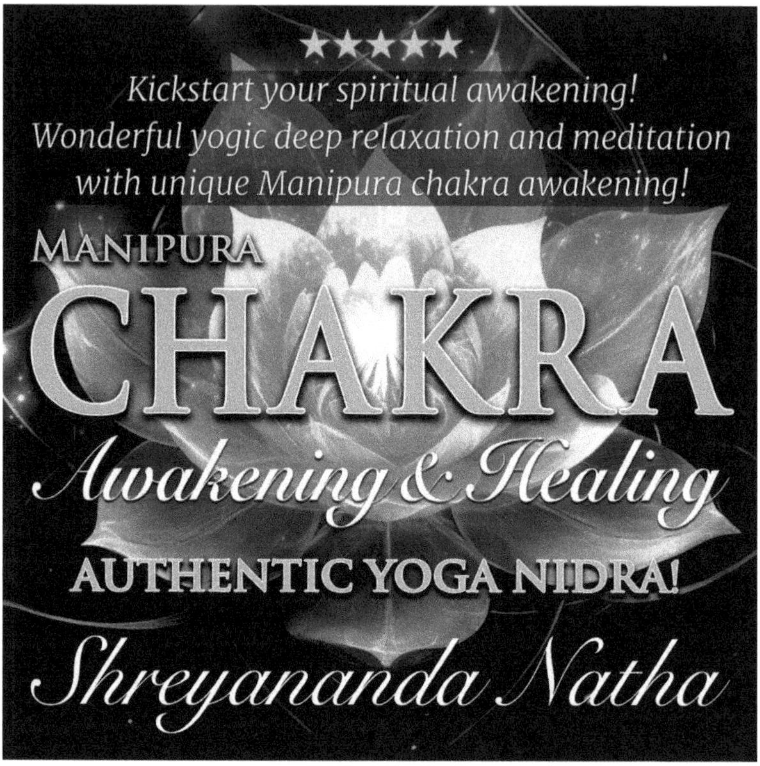

★ ★ ★ ★ ★
Kickstart your spiritual awakening!
Wonderful yogic deep relaxation and meditation
with unique Manipura chakra awakening!
MANIPURA
CHAKRA
Awakening & Healing
AUTHENTIC YOGA NIDRA!
Shreyananda Natha

www.ingramcontent.com/pod-product-compliance
Lightning Source LLC
LaVergne TN
LVHW051056180726
843512LV00019B/1498